Homemade Sunscreen

20 Natural Sun Lotions and After-Sun Moisturizer Recipes

Table of Contents

Introduction

Apart from direct effect the sun has on our health, it also makes us happier. You've probably noticed yourself that you smile more during summer than in cold winter days. There is a scientific explanation for this - UV rays stimulate the retina and the optic nerve centers of the brain, which then secretes increased serotonin - the most important hormone of happiness.

In just a few minutes sunlight makes us happy and relieves the fear. The beneficial effect of sun exposure is seen in reducing stress and regulating the immune system, cardiovascular and digestive organs.

The problem is, knowing when to stop. The fact is that the ozone layer is damaged, so the sun can be dangerous. To get all of the benefits from sunbathing, including a nice bronze tan, you need to pay special attention. One of the best ways to assure safe sun exposure is using sun protection lotions.

However, those found in markets might contain some chemicals that are far from being healthy. That is why we advise you to make your won and in this book we will provide you with the details on how to do it.

Chapter 1 – Homemade Sun Lotions vs. Commercial Lotions

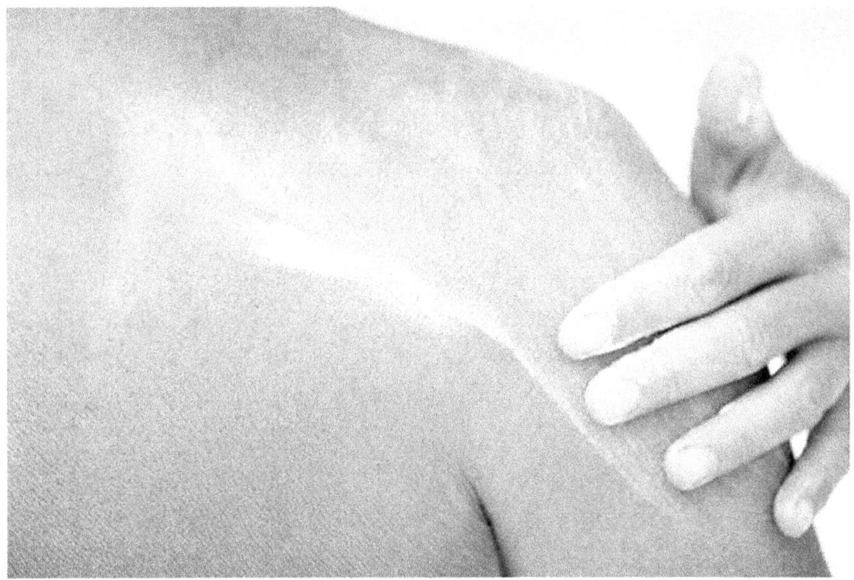

The fact is that 84 percent of sunscreens harmful to your health. The research was done by the EWG, one of the largest non-profit organizations in the United States. In most industrial sunscreen lotions a lot of toxic substances and chemicals that interfere with our endocrine system can be found.

The fact is that people are having a lot of skin problems even when they're using sun protection. In fact, since commercial sun screen lotions became a global thing, the number of skin cancer cases has increased.

Some studies have shown that the reason for that lies in the fact that sun lotions are responsible for increasing the number of free radicals – cells that are the main culprits for cancer and various other diseases.

Environmental Working Group (EWG) released the results of studies that found that 75 percent of 2,000 surveyed creams and lotions contain harmful chemicals that increase the risk of cancer and other diseases.

The research found that many of the ingredients of sun blocks and sunscreens get in the blood, some of which have toxic effects. Some of those release free radicals that damage the skin; others act as estrogen and disrupt the hormone balance. On top of that, some chemicals can cause allergic reactions and irritate the skin.

Bad news do not end there – most of the lotions examined contain chemicals that are known as substances that can cause cancer. Those include oxybenzone, methoxycinnamate, and PABA. If you take a look at the ingredients on your sun lotion, you might notice these ingredients, but some manufacturers decide to use codes as this area is not completely regulated by the law.

Another problem with commercial sun lotions is that over 30% of them contain nano-particles. Scientists from the CSIRO laboratories have proved that nano-particles of metal oxides can penetrate the skin cells and damage their DNA. Report from ABC (Australian Broadcasting Corporation) about the potential risks of using tanning lotion with SPF protection states that upon recently nanotechnology was considered a revolutionary technology, which helps the supply of clean water, removing viruses and bacteria, as well as increasing the durability of food.

Nano-science is also used for the production of clothing resistant to rain, creasing and stains, the skin aging and sunscreen products. However, since this technology is widely deployed, the question arose of whether the nano-particles are actually harmless to human health and the environment.

Scientists warn that young, too old or damaged skin can easily absorb nano-particles of titanium dioxide and zinc oxide, which many sunscreens contain. This means that there is a real danger that some of these particles can cause problems in your skin, which can lead to serious health issues. Because this area is still a new one, we can't be sure if the nano-particles are harmful, but it seems it's better to be safe, than sorry.

Why would you use products that have the potential to harm you, if you can make your own, totally safe lotions, made one hundred percent from natural ingredients? Homemade sun lotions can have the same factor of UV protection as those you get in stores, but with these you are absolutely sure they are healthy. On top of that, homemade sunscreens do not cost much, at least not as commercial ones.

The best thing about homemade sun lotions is that anyone can make them, because the ingredients needed are those found in your kitchen. Natural oils such as hazelnut are great for sun protection and should be the basic of your homemade sun lotion. This particular oil has the sun protection factor of 30. If you want an even better protection, think about buying the oil from raspberry seeds as its SPF is over 50.

Wheat germ oil is also a great option. This oil has the SPF of 20, but on top of that, it contains a really high amount of vitamin E, which is responsible for skin softness. If you use this oil, you can be certain your skin will get the bronze tan you wanted.

Other natural oils you can use as ingredients for your homemade sun lotion include the following:

- macadamia oil – SPF: 6

- sesame oil – SPF: 2 - 4

- coconut oil - SPF: 2 - 8

- olive oil - SPF: 2 - 8

- avocado oil SPF: - 4-15

- castor oil – SPF: 6

- almond oil – SPF: 5

Perhaps the best way would be to use as many of them as possible in the mixture, but apart from oils, you should also add other UV-protecting ingredients. Zinc oxide is a natural mineral which is great for protection from bad UV rays.

It is an antiseptic and has antifungal properties, which makes it great for using as a preservative in natural skin care lotions. Zinc oxide is usually added to the creams and lotions in the concentration of 2 to 10%.

Titanium dioxide is another mineral that has great properties related to skin car. It is often combined with zinc oxide. By adding up to five percent of the powder into the mixture, you will get the UV protection factor of at least 10.

Another substance you could add to the homemade lotion is Helioguard 365. The substance is an extract of red algae Porphyra umbilicalis, which is a very effective natural UVA filter. It is suitable for everyday use and protects the skin from premature aging.

To make it easier for you, we decided to provide you with 20 natural non-toxic sun lotions recipes, which are not expensive and are easy to make.

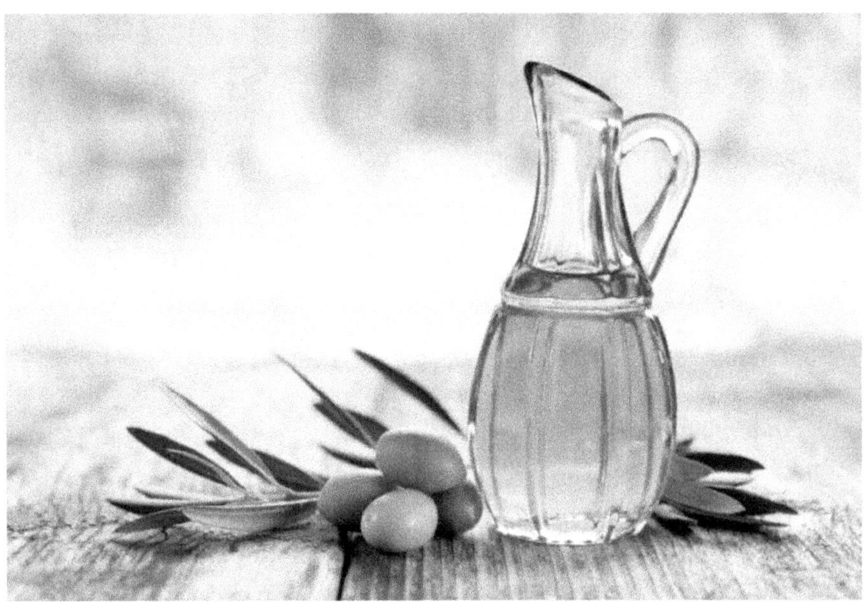

All of these sun lotions are one hundred percent safe and made of natural ingredients. They will make your skin look nice, enabling you to get bronze tan. On top of that, they will protect you from negative aspects of sunbathing.

Carrot Seed Oil Sunscreen

The base of this lotion is carrot seed oil, which has the sun protection factor of 40, which is capable of blocking 98% of ultraviolet rays. Apart from protecting your skin from dangerous rays, it also provides it with valuable vitamins and minerals. On top of that, this oil is very rich in antioxidants.

Ingredients:

- half a cup virgin olive oil

- ¼ cup carrot seed oil

- 2 teaspoons zinc oxide

- ¼ cup beeswax

Mix all of the ingredients apart from zinc oxide in a glass cup. Heat it up by putting the cup into hot water. Stir the mixture until you get a homogeneous blend. When done, let it cool off and add the zinc oxide.

Raspberry Seed Oil Lotion

Raspberry seed oil is one of the best UV-protectors found in nature. The SPF of this oil can be up to 50. Because of these and many other healthy properties, this oil could be expensive, so it is recommended to mix it with other oils.

Ingredients:

- 2 teaspoons raspberry seed oil

- Half a cup virgin olive oil

- ¼ cup coconut oil

- ¼ cup beeswax

As this mixture is very powerful for UV-protection, there's no need for adding zinc oxide, not any additional ingredients apart from those listed above. Simply mix all of these ingredients in a bowl and the lotion is ready.

Wheat Germ Oil Lotion

Wheat germ oil is very rich in vitamin E and other substances that are beneficial for skin health. You can even use it on its own as wheat germ oil has a very high sun protection factor.

Ingredients:

- 2 teaspoons wheat germ oil

- Half a cup virgin olive oil

- Two teaspoons almond oil

All of the ingredients are liquid, so all you have to do is mix them properly, before putting onto your skin.

Marigold Sunscreen

Marigold is known for having great effect on the skin, which is why it has been used in cosmetic since the antiquity. If you decide on using fresh marigold flowers, which is recommended, it would be good if you could leave the lotion to rest for at least a month, before using it.

Ingredients:

- 1 cup virgin olive oil

- half a carrot

- 2 teaspoons zinc oxide

- marigold flower

You need to use zinc oxide for this lotion, so bacteria wouldn't ruin it. Grate the carrot and add it to the oil, together with the rest of the ingredients. Leave it to rest for at least a couple of weeks at room temperature. When it's ready, strain it and put in a bottle, so you could carry it with you. If you wish the lotion to be thicker, feel free to add beeswax.

Avocado Oil Sunscreen Lotion

Avocado oil contains a large amount of mono-saturated fats, which are great for your skin. These substances will make your skin glow and help it fight dryness. On top of that, avocado oil has a pretty high SPF, which is 15.

Ingredients:

- ½ a cup avocado oil

- ½ a cup beeswax

- 2 teaspoons zinc oxide

Mix the oil with beeswax and place it in a glass container. Heat it up, so the two ingredients would mix nicely. When done, let it cool down and add zinc oxide.

Soybean Oil Cream

Chinese people use soybean oil for all sorts of things. Their traditional medicine known about good impact this oil has on skin for ages. You can use it to moisturize your skin, but this oil will also protect you from dangerous UV rays.

Ingredients:

- ½ a cup soybean oil

- ¼ cup shea butter

- ¼ cup coconut butter

- 2 tbsp. beeswax granules

Mix all of the ingredients in a bowl and keep on stirring until it becomes a homogenous mass.

Green Walnuts Sun Lotion

Leaving 5-6 green walnuts to stay in oil for a couple of weeks will make them release valuable ingredients, which are great for the health of your skin. Green walnuts are the most important ingredient in this lotion. Depending on your skin type you can choose the oils of different SPF.

Ingredients:

- 5-6 green walnuts

- 1 cup olive oil

- Teaspoon of avocado oil (or some other oil with high SPF)

Cut the walnuts into small pieces and put them in the oil. Let it rest for at least two weeks, before straining the oil and using it as a sun lotion.

Coconut Oil Sun Cream

You can use coconut oil for a variety of things, including cooking and greasing your hair. On top of that, this oil can be used for sun protection, because its sun protection factor is about 8.

Ingredients:

- ¼ cup coconut oil

- ¼ shea butter

- ¼ beeswax

- 1 teaspoon zinc oxide

Mix coconut oil, shea butter and beeswax in a bowl and heat it. Stir until you mix it well. When done, let it rest and add zinc oxide. The mixture should be a thick cream.

Macadamia Nut Oil Sun Lotion

Even on its own, macadamia oil is great for your skin. But, when you mix it with other oils, you will get an amazing sun protect lotion.

- ¼ cup macadamia oil

- ¼ cup sesame oil

- ¼ cup olive oil

- ¼ cup coconut oil

It is fairly easy to make this lotion. All you have to do is to mix all of the oils together and apply the mixture on your skin, afterwards.

Almond Oil Lotion

Although the sun protection factor of almond oil is just 5, this oil has a lot of other ingredients beneficial for your skin. Combine it with oils with higher SPF and you will get a very good sunscreen.

Ingredients:

- ¼ cup almond oil

- ¼ cup olive oil

- 2 teaspoons cup wheat germ oil

- 2 teaspoons castor oil

- 2 teaspoons avocado oil

- 1 teaspoon titanium dioxide

- 1 teaspoon zinc oxide

Pour all of these oils into a bowl and stir gently. Now add titanium dioxide and zinc oxide powder and your lotion is ready to go.

Jojoba Oil Lotion

Jojoba is great for your skin. It will make it moist and beautiful. On top of that, it can even help you fight stretch marks. Its SPF is not high, so you should mix it with other oils, which have higher sun protection factor.

Ingredients:

- ¼ cup jojoba oil

- ¼ cup hazelnut oil

- ¼ cup olive oil

- ¼ cup coconut oil

- 1 teaspoon zinc oxide

If you feel the lotion should be thicker, once you're done with stirring the mixture, you can add 2 teaspoon beeswax.

Myrrh Sun Protection Cream

Myrrh oil is a powerful antioxidant and contains substances that are great for your skin. On top of that, this oil can help you relax and sleep better.

However, its SPF is not very good. Because of that, you need to use other substances to make a sun cream.

Ingredients:

- 2 teaspoons myrrh oil

- ¼ cup hazelnut oil

- 2 teaspoons avocado oil

- 1 teaspoon titanium dioxide

- 1 teaspoon zinc oxide

- ¼ cup beeswax

First, you need to mix the oils together. It would be good if you did it at a higher temperature (but not boiling). When done, add the powder of titanium dioxide and zinc oxide. Finally, stir in the beeswax to make the mixture thick.

Lavender Sun Lotion

Lavender is a plant that has properties good for your skin. Although, it is not good in keeping you protected from UV rays, it can help with sunburns. Prevention is the key, so you can use lavender lotion when going to sunbath, under condition that it contains oils with high SPF.

- 1 teaspoon lavender oil

- ¼ cup hazelnut oil

- 2 teaspoons avocado oil

- 1 teaspoon titanium dioxide

- 1 teaspoon zinc oxide

- ¼ cup beeswax

Mix beeswax and the oils in a glass bowl. Place the bowl into hot water, so the mixture would become homogenous. At the end, add zinc and titanium powder.

Waterproof Chamomile Sunscreen

Chamomile is a plant that has been used in cosmetics for ages. It is knows to have the ability to cam irritated skin, so you should think about making a sunscreen that contains this plant.

- 1 cup chamomile tea

- 1 teaspoon lavender oil

- ¼ cup hazelnut oil

- 2 teaspoons avocado oil

- 1 teaspoon zinc oxide

Put the chamomile tea in the mixture of all the oils listed above. Leave it there for a couple of days, before straining the oil. The final step is adding 1 teaspoon of zinc oxide in the lotion.

Whipped Shea Butter Cream

Sun protection factor of this cream can be above 50. That is why you can use it to protect your face.

Ingredients:

- 1/2 cup Shea Butter

- 1/3 cup Coconut oil

- 1 teaspoon carrot seed essential oil

- 1 teaspoon myrrh essential oil

- 1 teaspoon zinc oxide

Put all of the ingredients in a bowl and whip it until you get a thick cream.

Aloe Vera Sunscreen Lotion

This is a liquid lotion, which you can put into a sprayer bottle. The SPF of the lotion should be above 20.

Ingredients:

- 1 cup aloe vera juice

- 1 teaspoon lavender oil

- ¼ cup hazelnut oil

- 2 teaspoons avocado oil

There isn't too much hustle to make this lotion. Simply mix all of the ingredients together and pour the mixture into a sprayer bottle.

Helioguard 365 Sunscreen

Helioguard 365 is one of the bets substances you can get for your skin. We recommend using it in a mixture with certain high-SPF oils to create a perfect sun lotion.

- Helioguard 365 extract

- ¼ cup shea butter

- 1/8 cup coconut oil

- 1/8 cup olive oil

- 1 teaspoon beeswax

Simply put all of the ingredients and whip it until you create a cream.

Snow Algae Sun Lotion

One of the cons of regular sunbathing is that it dries the skin and makes it age faster. The solution lies in using proper lotions, such as this one, in which the key ingredient is snow algae powder.

Ingredients:

- 1 teaspoon snow algae powder

- ¼ cup hazelnut oil

- 2 teaspoons avocado oil

- 1 teaspoon titanium dioxide

- 1 teaspoon zinc oxide

- ¼ cup beeswax

Pour all of these oils into a bowl and stir gently. Now add titanium dioxide and zinc oxide powder and your lotion is complete.

Essential Oils Sunscreen

If we had to rank top three essential oils for skin, our pick would be lavender, geranium and basil. Combined with oils with high SPF, this lotion is all you need to look beautiful.

Ingredients:

- 10 drops lavender essential oil

- 10 drops geranium essential oil

- 10 drops basil essential oil

- ½ a cup olive oil

- ¼ cup hazelnut oil

- 1 teaspoon zinc oxide

Making this lotion doesn't require much effort – simply mix all of the ingredients together.

Black Tea Sunscreen

Tea plant is known for treating aging skin and fighting fungal infections. Because it helps with skin moisturizing, it can be used in sun lotions, of course only combined with ingredients with high SPF.

Ingredients:

- 1 teaspoon black tea leaves

- ¼ cup soybean oil

- ¼ wheat germ oil

- ¼ hazelnut oil

- 1 teaspoon zinc oxide

- 1teaspoon titanium dioxide

- 1/8 cup beeswax

Grind black tea leaves until you get fine powder. Mix it with the rest of the ingredients and apply on the skin.

Chapter 3 – Why to use After-Sun Lotions?

After each sunbathing, it is advisable to use lotions that will cool your skin and help with inflammatory processes if any occur. On top of that, these lotions have properties that can regenerate the skin. After-sun lotions should contain antioxidants which neutralize the effect of free radicals, thus preventing cell damaging. Because of this, after-sun lotions will help your skin stay beautiful and healthy.

Using after-sun lotions will ensure your skin will not scale down, so the bronze tan will stay longer. However, apart from making your skin look beautiful, certain ingredients in these lotions can also help controlling the damage that might happen due to long exposure to UV rays.

Even if you don't get sunburn, you should use after-sun lotions anyway. In this case, after-sun lotions will act as regular lotions, moisturizing your skin. The problem occurs when you visit a drugstore to find an after-sun lotion. Buying a random one could be risky, because you don't know which substances manufacturers use. If you want to find a perfect, natural solution, you will probably have to spend a lot of money.

Because of all the reasons mentioned above, we advise you to stay away from buying any kind of commercial after-sun lotions, not only those cheap ones.

To stay safe and to spare your money, the best solution is to make your own lotion.

Making a lotion in your own home is not a rocket science. All you need is a bowl and certain ingredients, which you might already have in your kitchen. By using only natural ingredients, you will be sure nothing bad could happen to your skin. On top of that, if you properly make them, your skin will stay beautiful for a long period of time.

Chapter 4 – After-Sun Moisturizer Recipes

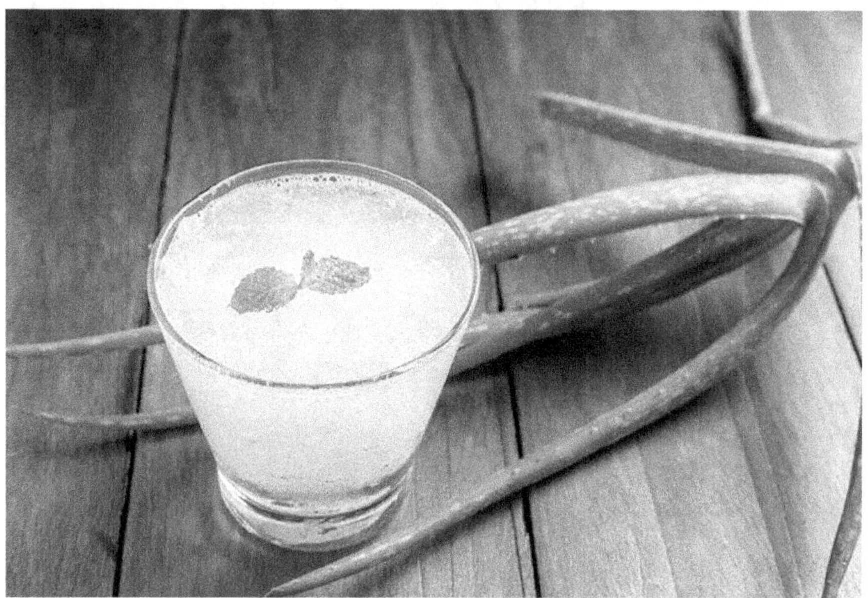

It is inevitable that your skin will become dry if you spend time exposed to direct sunshine. Instead of getting away from it, you need to embrace the sun and look for other solutions.

The best solution is to use after-sun lotions. We present you with a few recipes for after-sun moisturizers, which will make your skin glow and help if there's any burning or itching.

Aloe Vera After-Sun Moisturizer

Aloe vera is a super plant when it comes to skin issues. Using the extract from this plant will surely help your skin stay moisturized. On top of that, it will prevent the burnt skin layers from peeling off. This lotion also contains other ingrains that are also great for skin care.

Ingredients:

- 1 cup aloe vera juice

- ½ cup coconut oil

- 1 teaspoon chamomile extract

- ¼ cup beeswax

Simply mix all of the ingredients in a bowl and place it in the fridge before you go out in the sun. The cold lotion will make you feel great when you apply it on your hot skin.

After-Sun Yogurt Cream

For centuries people have been using Greek yogurt as a way of curing skin problems. It is a fact that yogurt is great moisturizer, but when you add certain essential oils to it, the mixture becomes a superb after sun cream.

Ingredients:

- ½ cup Greek yogurt

- 1 teaspoon cup sesame oil

- ¼ cup shea butter

Mix all of the ingredients and put them in the freezer to cool. Apply on your skin right after sunbathing.

Essential Oils After-Sun Moisturizer

Essential oils help regeneration of your skin, helping it fighting with sunburns and dryness. Because of these properties, it is wise to apply them onto your skin after a long exposure to direct sunshine. However, essential oils also help your skin stay hydrated and can slow down the aging process. That is why you can use this lotion even when it's not summer.

Ingredients:

- 10 drops lavender essential oil

- 10 drops geranium essential oil

- 10 drops basil essential oil

- ½ a cup olive oil

- ¼ cup hazelnut oil

- ¼ cup aloe vera juice

Using Sunscreens as After-Sun Moisturizers

Oils used for making sun protection lotions have properties that will moisturize your skin. So, basically, you can use any kind of oil for this purpose, from olive and coconut oil, to carrot seed oil.

The only thing you should avoid using is zinc oxide. This means that when making homemade sunscreens, you can make after-sun lotions from the same ingredients.

Here is a list that can help you to decide which oils to use for your after-sun moisturizing lotion:

- Basil essential oil

- Lavender essential oil

- Geranium essential oil

- Frankincense essential oil

- Ylang Ylang essential oil

- Lemongrass essential oil

- Rose essential oil

- Tea tree essential oil

- Carrot seed oil

- Jojoba oil

- Coconut oil

- Avocado oil

- Almond oil

- Sea buckthorn berry oil

- Neroli oil

- Cypress oil

- Olive oil

Chapter 5 – How to Make Homemade Tan Activators?

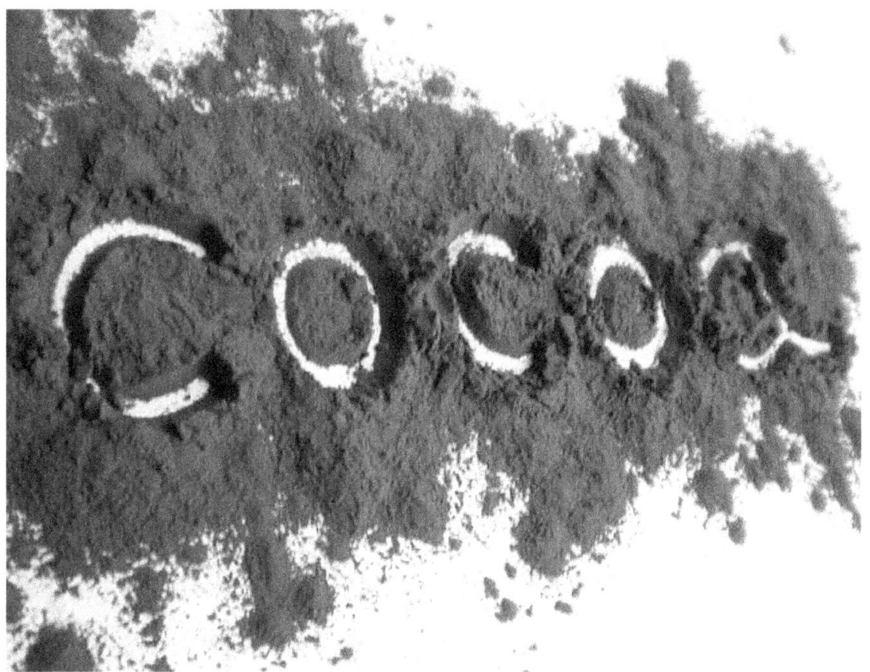

Sometimes you don't have enough time to spend on sunbathing, but you still want to have beautiful tan. You don't have to worry as there's a solution for you.

Using a homemade tan activator is a great way to get a tan, without exposing your skin to dangerous UV rays for too long.

On top of that, even if you stay long in the sun, you can use these lotions as they will make your skin even more beautiful and will make your bronze tan last longer.

Ingredients:

- 2 teaspoons carrot seed oil

- 10 drops Helioguard 365 extract

- ¼ cup almond oil

- ¼ cup aloe vera juice

- ¼ cup coconut oil

- ¼ cup pure cocoa powder

Each of these ingredients has amazing properties great for your skin. On top of that, certain substances found here are known as tan activators, which means that you will get a great tan, even if you spend only a few minutes exposed to direct sun.

On top of that, cocoa powder will act as natural dye, giving you an instant tanned look.

Instead of cocoa, you can use black tea. Some people also find that coffee works for them.

The truth is that different skin types react differently to certain substances, so what is good for one person might not be the perfect solution for another. Another factor is what you want to get from the tan activators, that is, how tanned you want to get.

For getting a nice tan, you might also want to think about modifying your diet a bit as it can have a great impact on your skin. For a few weeks before the summer, you should start eating more foods that are rich in beta-carotene. Those include carrots and green leafy vegetables.

Omega fatty acids are also very important for the skin health, so start munching on seeds and nuts as well. In fact, a healthy lifestyle and a healthy diet could be the key to beautiful tan.

Conclusion

Having a nice tan certainly makes you look healthier and more attractive. In fact, researches have shown that people with tanned skin look leaner than those with the same weight but pale skin. Because of all this, getting a nice tan has become such a big thing in the world, especially among young people, who are not aware of the dangers of extensive sunbathing.

Apart from problems direct exposure to sunlight causes straight away, such as burning sensation or itching of the skin, it can have way more serious consequences. Skin cancer is the number one reason why people want to stay away from the sun, but hiding in the dark is equally dangerous.

In fact, it is suggested that more people get cancer from not being exposed to sun. That said, sunbathing can be very healthy for you, but only if done properly.

The best way to get a nice tan, while not risking your health is to use sunscreens. But again a problem rises as commercial lotions might be full of poison. That is why we can't stress how important is to make your own sunscreen lotions.

In this book you've seen that making them is not that hard. Most of the things you need might already be in your kitchen. If not, you can easily get them in the stores, without spending too much money.

Apart from homemade sunscreens, this book showed you how to make after-sun lotions, which will help your bronze tan last longer. On top of that, these lotions can be used on regular basis as organic moisturizers that help the skin stay young.

Finally, we showed you a trick which can help you get a nice tan in a short period of time. By making your own tan activator, you will help your skin stay tanned for a longer period, while not putting burning it on sun.

The best thing about all of the lotions mentioned in this book is that they are one hundred percent natural and completely safe, which means you can use them all the time, not only during the hottest summer months.

Keeping in touch with nature is the key for a healthy life and using organic sun lotions certainly can't harm you.

FREE Bonus Reminder

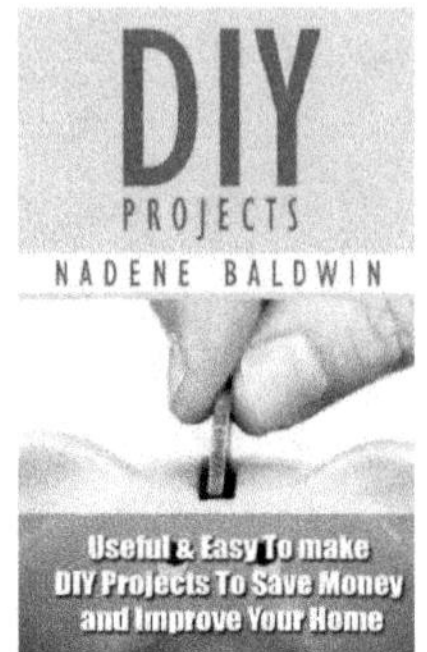

If you have not grabbed it yet, please go ahead and download your special bonus report *"DIY Projects. 13 Useful & Easy To Make DIY Projects To Save Money & Improve Your Home!"*

Simply Click the Button Below

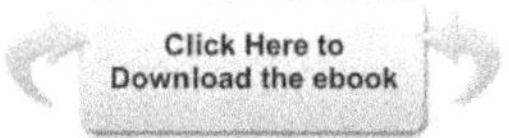

OR **Go to This Page**

http://diyhomecraft.com/free

BONUS #2: More Free & Discounted Books

Do you want to receive more Free & Discounted Books?

We have a mailing list where we send out our new Books when they go free or with a discount on Kindle. Click on the link below to sign up for Free & Discount Book Promotions.

=> Sign Up for Free & Discount Book Promotions <=

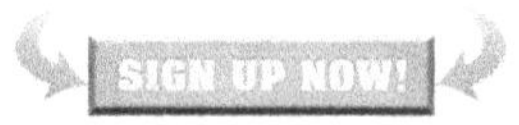

OR Go to this URL

http://zbit.ly/1WBb1Ek